THE CHRISTIAN NURSES & *Caregivers* JOURNAL

Devotional Journal & Self-Care Planner

Thank You

FROM THE CHRISTIAN *Nurses & Caregivers* JOURNAL

Thank you for purchasing this Christian Nurses and Caregivers Journal. We pray this is a blessing to those who give so much and need help to find spaces for quiet time and self-care, and to connect with the God who cares for them.

Be sure to check out our other titles, including journals for Christian:

- Creatives of all kinds
- Praise and Worship Leaders, Singers, and Choir Members
- Musicians
- Fashion Designers
- Interior Designers and more...

Look for us at:

- Purposehousepublishing.com
- Etsy
- TikTok

The Christian *Nurses and Caregivers*

Devotional Journal & Self-Care Planner

Because God Cares for the Caregiver

This Journal Belongs To:

____

From:

____

Date:

____

Published by PurposeHouse Publishing, Columbia, Maryland. Cover Design by PurposeHouse Publishing (www.purposehousepublishing.com). Printed in the USA.

ISBN: 978-1-957190-45-7

THE CHRISTIAN NURSES & *Caregivers* JOURNAL

Devotional Journal & Self-Care Planner

SCRIPTURE MEDITATIONS AND REFLECTIONS, SHIFT SCHEDULE AND NOTES PAGES, DAILY TO-DOS, AND WEEKLY SELF-CARE PLANNING

Lenita Reeves

Purpose House Publishing

HOW TO USE THIS CHRISTIAN NURSES & *Caregivers* JOURNAL

A perfect gift for a nurse, caregiver, or doctor, this pocket-sized Scripture journal and planner fits perfectly in lab jackets' or scrubs' pockets. Each of its Scriptures focuses on God's love and care for the caregiver, refueling the spiritual tank of those who give so much of themselves each day.

The first day of the week begins with a weekly Scripture meditation, followed by weekly "care-casting", gratitude, scheduling, and self-care planning.

Then, the following six days of the week each have a daily Scripture journal page and a page for daily shift notes and to-dos.

The journal covers 4 complete weeks, with the 5th week being 3 days (31 days total) to facilitate any month of the year.

HOW TO USE THIS CHRISTIAN NURSES & Caregivers JOURNAL

Each week includes a weekly:

- Scripture meditation page (Day 1 of the week)
- Reflection page with space to respond to the meditation
- Care-casting page, including coworkers and patients you are giving to the Lord and space to note your weekly self-care goal
- Shift schedule page
- Self-care evaluation page
- Self-care planning page for the next week

Each of the remaining six days of the week has a:

- Scripture journal page
- Shift notes and to-do's page

This is wonderful tool to journal and have quiet time with the Lord and remind yourself of His care for you as you work.

New Week
Scripture Meditation

For The Week Beginning / /
Day 1 of Week 1

Since God cares for you, let Him carry all your burdens and worries.
- 1 Peter 5:7 Voice

Visualize the verse(s). What do the verse(s) speak to you, what emotions or memories do they invoke? What story do they tell or remind you of? What is God saying to you through the Scripture(s), and what can you speak back to Him?

This Week's Prayer & Reflection

For The Week Beginning / /
Day 1 of the Week

Heavenly Father, today, the first day of my week, I think of your care for me. I place my week into your caring hands.

Since God cares for you, let Him carry all your burdens and worries. - 1 Peter 5:7 Voice

This Week: In the Father's Care

Since God cares for you, let Him carry all your burdens and worries. - 1 Peter 5:7 Voice

Cares I'm Casting This Week

Coworker I'm Praying For

Patient I'm Praying For

I'm Grateful For

This Week's Shift Schedule

For The Week Beginning / /

Sunday
Monday
Tuesday
Wednesday
Thursday
Friday
Saturday

To Dos

- [ ] ______________
- [ ] ______________
- [ ] ______________
- [ ] ______________
- [ ] ______________
- [ ] ______________
- [ ] ______________
- [ ] ______________

Weekly Self-Care Goal

One "self-care" thing I can do this week is . . .

Daily Scripture & Prayer

Date / /

Deuteronomy 32:9-10 NIV: For the Lord's portion is his people, Jacob his allotted inheritance. [10] In a desert land he found him, in a barren and howling waste. He shielded him and cared for him; he guarded him as the apple of his eye.

Thank you for peace. Thank you for protection. Thank you for patience for my patients.

...day's Reminders & Shift Notes

Shift Notes

To Dos

- [ ]
- [ ]
- [ ]
- [ ]
- [ ]
- [ ]
- [ ]
- [ ]
- [ ]
- [ ]
- [ ]
- [ ]

Daily Scripture & Prayer

Date / /

Job 10:12 NKJV: You have granted me life and favor, And Your care has preserved my spirit.

Thank you for peace. Thank you for protection. Thank you for patience for my patients.

Today's Reminders & Shift Notes

Shift Notes

To Dos

Daily Scripture & Prayer

Date / /

Psalm 27:10 NKJV: When my father and my mother forsake me, Then the Lord will take care of me.

Thank you for peace. Thank you for protection. Thank you for patience for my patients.

Today's Reminders & Shift Notes

Shift Notes

To Dos

Daily Scripture & Prayer

Date / /

Psalm 55:22 NIV: Cast your cares on the Lord and he will sustain you; he will never let the righteous be shaken

Thank you for peace. Thank you for protection. Thank you for patience for my patients.

Today's Reminders & Shift Notes

Shift Notes

To Dos

Daily Scripture & Prayer

Date / /

Psalm 95:6-7 NIV: Come, let us bow down in worship, let us kneel before the Lord our Maker;
7 for he is our God and we are the people of his pasture, the flock under his care.

Thank you for peace. Thank you for protection. Thank you for patience for my patients.

Today's Reminders & Shift Notes

Shift Notes

To Dos

Daily Scripture & Prayer

Date / /

Jeremiah 15:15 NIV: Lord, you understand; remember me and care for me. Avenge me on my persecutors. You are long-suffering—do not take me away; think of how I suffer reproach for your sake.

Thank you for peace. Thank you for protection. Thank you for patience for my patients.

Today's Reminders & Shift Notes

Shift Notes

To Dos

- [ ]
- [ ]
- [ ]
- [ ]
- [ ]
- [ ]
- [ ]
- [ ]
- [ ]
- [ ]
- [ ]
- [ ]

This Week's Self-Care

Daily Scripture Meditation and quiet time with God is a form of self-care. Here are other kinds of self-care to evaluate this week. You'll set goals for next week on the next page.

Basic Needs

This week I got enough:

- ☐ Sleep
- ☐ Nutritious Food
- ☐ Physical Activity
- ☐ Personal Hygiene

Weekly Self-Care Goal

I met my weekly self-care goal this week:

- ☐ Yes
- ☐ No

Other Needs

This week I got enough:

- ☐ Social Interaction (investing in healthy relationships)
- ☐ Mental Stimulation/Exercise (puzzles, reading, creative activity)
- ☐ Emotional Balance (dealing with anger, anxiety, or other emotions)

Next Week's Self-Care Areas to Improve

Check the areas to improve next week:

Basic Needs

- ☐ Sleep
- ☐ Nutritious Food
- ☐ Physical Activity
- ☐ Personal Hygiene

Other Needs

- ☐ Social Interaction
(investing in healthy relationships)
- ☐ Mental Stimulation/Exercise
(puzzles, reading, creative activity)
- ☐ Emotional Balance
(dealing with anger, anxiety, or other emotions)
- ☐ Other: ______________________

New Week
Scripture Meditation

For The Week Beginning / /
Day 1 of Week 2

Nahum 1:7 NIV: The Lord is good, a refuge in times of trouble. He cares for those who trust in him.

Visualize the verse(s). What do the verse(s) speak to you, what emotions or memories do they invoke? What story do they tell or remind you of? What is God saying to you through the Scripture(s), and what can you speak back to Him?

This Week's Prayer & Reflection

For The Week Beginning / /
Day 1 of the Week

Heavenly Father, today, the first day of my week, I think of your care for me. I place my week into your caring hands.

Nahum 1:7 NIV: The Lord is good, a refuge in times of trouble. He cares for those who trust in him.

This Week: In the Father's Care

Nahum 1:7 NIV: The Lord is good, a refuge in times of trouble. He cares for those who trust in him.

Cares I'm Casting This Week

Coworker I'm Praying For

Patient I'm Praying For

I'm Grateful For

This Week's Shift Schedule

For The Week Beginning / /

Sunday
Monday
Tuesday
Wednesday
Thursday
Friday
Saturday

To Dos

- [ ] ____________________
- [ ] ____________________
- [ ] ____________________
- [ ] ____________________
- [ ] ____________________
- [ ] ____________________
- [ ] ____________________
- [ ] ____________________

Weekly Self-Care Goal

One "self-care" thing I can do this week is . . .

Daily Scripture & Prayer

Date / /

Hosea 13:4-5 NIV: "But I have been the Lord your God ever since you came out of Egypt. You shall acknowledge no God but me, no Savior except me. [5] I cared for you in the wilderness, in the land of burning heat.

Thank you for peace. Thank you for protection. Thank you for patience for my patients.

Today's Reminders & Shift Notes

Shift Notes

To Dos

Daily Scripture & Prayer

Date / /

Luke 4:10 NIV: For it is written: "'He will command his angels concerning you to guard you carefully.

Thank you for peace. Thank you for protection. Thank you for patience for my patients.

Today's Reminders & Shift Notes

Shift Notes

To Dos

- [ ]
- [ ]
- [ ]
- [ ]
- [ ]
- [ ]
- [ ]
- [ ]
- [ ]
- [ ]
- [ ]
- [ ]

Daily Scripture & Prayer

Date / /

John 10:12,14-15 NIV: The hired hand is not the shepherd and does not own the sheep. [14] "I am the good shepherd; I know my sheep and my sheep know me— [15] just as the Father knows me and I know the Father—and I lay down my life for the sheep.

Thank you for peace. Thank you for protection. Thank you for patience for my patients.

Today's Reminders & Shift Notes

Shift Notes

To Dos

Daily Scripture & Prayer

Date / /

Philippians 4:6-7 NIV: Be careful for nothing; but in every thing by prayer and supplication with thanksgiving let your requests be made known unto God. 7 And the peace of God, which passeth all understanding, shall keep your hearts and minds through Christ Jesus.

Thank you for peace. Thank you for protection. Thank you for patience for my patients.

Today's Reminders & Shift Notes

Shift Notes	To Dos

Daily Scripture & Prayer

Date / /

Deuteronomy 31:8 NIV: The Lord himself goes before you and will be with you; he will never leave you nor forsake you. Do not be afraid; do not be discouraged."

Thank you for peace. Thank you for protection. Thank you for patience for my patients.

Today's Reminders & Shift Notes

Shift Notes	To Dos

Daily Scripture & Prayer

Date / /

Matthew 11:28 NIV: "Come to me, all you who are weary and burdened, and I will give you rest.

Thank you for peace. Thank you for protection. Thank you for patience for my patients.

Today's Reminders & Shift Notes

Shift Notes

To Dos

This Week's Self-Care

Daily Scripture Meditation and quiet time with God is a form of self-care. Here are other kinds of self-care to evaluate this week. You'll set goals for next week on the next page.

Basic Needs

This week I got enough:

- ☐ Sleep
- ☐ Nutritious Food
- ☐ Physical Activity
- ☐ Personal Hygiene

Weekly Self-Care Goal

I met my weekly self-care goal this week:

- ☐ Yes
- ☐ No

Other Needs

This week I got enough:

- ☐ Social Interaction (investing in healthy relationships)
- ☐ Mental Stimulation/Exercise (puzzles, reading, creative activity)
- ☐ Emotional Balance (dealing with anger, anxiety, or other emotions)

Next Week's Self-Care Areas to Improve

Check the areas to improve next week:

Basic Needs

- ☐ Sleep
- ☐ Nutritious Food
- ☐ Physical Activity
- ☐ Personal Hygiene

Other Needs

- ☐ Social Interaction
  (investing in healthy relationships)
- ☐ Mental Stimulation/Exercise
  (puzzles, reading, creative activity)
- ☐ Emotional Balance
  (dealing with anger, anxiety, or other emotions)
- ☐ Other:______________________

New Week
Scripture Meditation

For The Week Beginning / /
Day 1 of Week 3

Isaiah 46:4 NIV: Even to your old age and gray hairs I am he, I am he who will sustain you. I have made you and I will carry you; I will sustain you and I will rescue you.

Visualize the verse(s). What do the verse(s) speak to you, what emotions or memories do they invoke? What story do they tell or remind you of? What is God saying to you through the Scripture(s), and what can you speak back to Him?

This Week's Prayer & Reflection

For The Week Beginning   /   /

Day 1 of the Week

Heavenly Father, today, the first day of my week, I think of your care for me. I place my week into your caring hands.

Isaiah 46:4 NIV: Even to your old age and gray hairs I am he, I am he who will sustain you. I have made you and I will carry you; I will sustain you and I will rescue you.

This Week: In the Father's Care

Isaiah 46:4 NIV: Even to your old age and gray hairs I am he, I am he who will sustain you. I have made you and I will carry you; I will sustain you and I will rescue you.

Cares I'm Casting This Week

Coworker I'm Praying For

Patient I'm Praying For

I'm Grateful For

This Week's Shift Schedule

For The Week Beginning / /

Day	
Sunday	
Monday	
Tuesday	
Wednesday	
Thursday	
Friday	
Saturday	

To Dos

- ☐ ______________
- ☐ ______________
- ☐ ______________
- ☐ ______________
- ☐ ______________
- ☐ ______________
- ☐ ______________
- ☐ ______________

Weekly Self-Care Goal

One "self-care" thing I can do this week is . . .

Daily Scripture & Prayer

Date / /

Matthew 6:31-33 NIV: So do not worry, saying, 'What shall we eat?' or 'What shall we drink?' or 'What shall we wear?' 32 For the pagans run after all these things, and your heavenly Father knows that you need them. 33 But seek first his kingdom and his righteousness, and all these things will be given to you as well.

Thank you for peace. Thank you for protection. Thank you for patience for my patients.

Today's Reminders & Shift Notes

Shift Notes

To Dos

Daily Scripture & Prayer

Date / /

Psalm 8:4 NIV: What is mankind that you are mindful of them, human beings that you care for them?

Thank you for peace. Thank you for protection. Thank you for patience for my patients.

Today's Reminders & Shift Notes

Shift Notes

To Dos

- [ ]
- [ ]
- [ ]
- [ ]
- [ ]
- [ ]
- [ ]
- [ ]
- [ ]
- [ ]
- [ ]
- [ ]

Daily Scripture & Prayer

Date / /

1 John 4:9-10 NIV: This is how God showed his love among us: He sent his one and only Son into the world that we might live through him. [10] This is love: not that we loved God, but that he loved us and sent his Son as an atoning sacrifice for our sins.

Thank you for peace. Thank you for protection. Thank you for patience for my patients.

Today's Reminders & Shift Notes

Shift Notes

To Dos

Daily Scripture & Prayer

Date / /

Matthew 10:29-31 NIV: Are not two sparrows sold for a penny? Yet not one of them will fall to the ground outside your Father's care. 30 And even the very hairs of your head are all numbered. 31 So don't be afraid; you are worth more than many sparrows.

Thank you for peace. Thank you for protection. Thank you for patience for my patients.

Today's Reminders & Shift Notes

Shift Notes

To Dos

Daily Scripture & Prayer

Date / /

Romans 8:38-39 NIV: For I am convinced that neither death nor life, neither angels nor demons, neither the present nor the future, nor any powers, 39 neither height nor depth, nor anything else in all creation, will be able to separate us from the love of God that is in Christ Jesus our Lord.

Thank you for peace. Thank you for protection. Thank you for patience for my patients.

Today's Reminders & Shift Notes

Shift Notes

To Dos

- [ ]
- [ ]
- [ ]
- [ ]
- [ ]
- [ ]
- [ ]
- [ ]
- [ ]
- [ ]
- [ ]
- [ ]

Daily Scripture & Prayer

Date / /

Philippians 4:19 NIV: And my God will meet all your needs according to the riches of his glory in Christ Jesus.

Thank you for peace. Thank you for protection. Thank you for patience for my patients.

Today's Reminders & Shift Notes

Shift Notes

To Dos

This Week's Self-Care

Daily Scripture Meditation and quiet time with God is a form of self-care. Here are other kinds of self-care to evaluate this week. You'll set goals for next week on the next page.

Basic Needs

This week I got enough:

- [ ] Sleep
- [ ] Nutritious Food
- [ ] Physical Activity
- [ ] Personal Hygiene

Weekly Self-Care Goal

I met my weekly self-care goal this week:

- [ ] Yes
- [ ] No

Other Needs

This week I got enough:

- [ ] Social Interaction (investing in healthy relationships)
- [ ] Mental Stimulation/Exercise (puzzles, reading, creative activity)
- [ ] Emotional Balance (dealing with anger, anxiety, or other emotions)

Next Week's Self-Care Areas to Improve

Check the areas to improve next week:

Basic Needs

- ☐ Sleep
- ☐ Nutritious Food
- ☐ Physical Activity
- ☐ Personal Hygiene

Other Needs

- ☐ Social Interaction (investing in healthy relationships)
- ☐ Mental Stimulation/Exercise (puzzles, reading, creative activity)
- ☐ Emotional Balance (dealing with anger, anxiety, or other emotions)
- ☐ Other: ______________________

New Week
Scripture Meditation

For The Week Beginning / /
Day 1 of Week 4

Isaiah 41:10 NIV: So do not fear, for I am with you; do not be dismayed, for I am your God. I will strengthen you and help you; I will uphold you with my righteous right hand.

Visualize the verse(s). What do the verse(s) speak to you, what emotions or memories do they invoke? What story do they tell or remind you of? What is God saying to you through the Scripture(s), and what can you speak back to Him?

This Week's Prayer & Reflection

For The Week Beginning / /

Day 1 of the Week

Heavenly Father, today, the first day of my week, I think of your care for me. I place my week into your caring hands.

Isaiah 41:10 NIV: So do not fear, for I am with you; do not be dismayed, for I am your God. I will strengthen you and help you; I will uphold you with my righteous right hand.

This Week: In the Father's Care

Isaiah 41:10 NIV: So do not fear, for I am with you; do not be dismayed, for I am your God. I will strengthen you and help you; I will uphold you with my righteous right hand.

Cares I'm Casting This Week

Coworker I'm Praying For

Patient I'm Praying For

I'm Grateful For

This Week's Shift Schedule

For The Week Beginning / /

Sunday
Monday
Tuesday
Wednesday
Thursday
Friday
Saturday

To Dos

- [ ] ____________
- [ ] ____________
- [ ] ____________
- [ ] ____________
- [ ] ____________
- [ ] ____________
- [ ] ____________
- [ ] ____________

Weekly Self-Care Goal

One "self-care" thing I can do this week is . . .

Daily Scripture & Prayer

Date / /

John 16:33 NIV: "I have told you these things, so that in me you may have peace. In this world you will have trouble. But take heart! I have overcome the world."

Thank you for peace. Thank you for protection. Thank you for patience for my patients.

Today's Reminders & Shift Notes

Shift Notes

To Dos

- [ ]
- [ ]
- [ ]
- [ ]
- [ ]
- [ ]
- [ ]
- [ ]
- [ ]
- [ ]
- [ ]
- [ ]

Daily Scripture & Prayer

Date / /

John 15:9 NIV: “As the Father has loved me, so have I loved you. Now remain in my love.

Thank you for peace. Thank you for protection. Thank you for patience for my patients.

Today's Reminders & Shift Notes

Shift Notes

To Dos

Daily Scripture & Prayer

Date / /

Romans 8:28 NIV: And we know that in all things God works for the good of those who love him, who[a] have been called according to his purpose.

Thank you for peace. Thank you for protection. Thank you for patience for my patients.

Today's Reminders & Shift Notes

Shift Notes	To Dos

Daily Scripture & Prayer

Date / /

Romans 5:8 NIV: But God demonstrates his own love for us in this: While we were still sinners, Christ died for us.

Thank you for peace. Thank you for protection. Thank you for patience for my patients.

Today's Reminders & Shift Notes

Shift Notes

To Dos

- [ ]
- [ ]
- [ ]
- [ ]
- [ ]
- [ ]
- [ ]
- [ ]
- [ ]
- [ ]
- [ ]
- [ ]

Daily Scripture & Prayer

Date / /

Psalm 91:4 NIV: He will cover you with his feathers, and under his wings you will find refuge; his faithfulness will be your shield and rampart.

Thank you for peace. Thank you for protection. Thank you for patience for my patients.

Today's Reminders & Shift Notes

Shift Notes

To Dos

Daily Scripture & Prayer

Date / /

Isaiah 43:1-2 NIV: But now, this is what the Lord says—he who created you, Jacob, he who formed you, Israel: "Do not fear, for I have redeemed you; I have summoned you by name; you are mine. [2] When you pass through the waters, I will be with you; and when you pass through the rivers, they will not sweep over you. When you walk through the fire, you will not be burned; the flames will not set you ablaze.

Thank you for peace. Thank you for protection. Thank you for patience for my patients.

Today's Reminders & Shift Notes

Shift Notes

To Dos

This Week's Self-Care

Daily Scripture Meditation and quiet time with God is a form of self-care. Here are other kinds of self-care to evaluate this week. You'll set goals for next week on the next page.

Basic Needs

This week I got enough:

- ☐ Sleep
- ☐ Nutritious Food
- ☐ Physical Activity
- ☐ Personal Hygiene

Weekly Self-Care Goal

I met my weekly self-care goal this week:

- ☐ Yes
- ☐ No

Other Needs

This week I got enough:

- ☐ Social Interaction (investing in healthy relationships)
- ☐ Mental Stimulation/Exercise (puzzles, reading, creative activity)
- ☐ Emotional Balance (dealing with anger, anxiety, or other emotions)

Next Week's Self-Care Areas to Improve

Check the areas to improve next week:

Basic Needs

- ☐ Sleep
- ☐ Nutritious Food
- ☐ Physical Activity
- ☐ Personal Hygiene

Other Needs

- ☐ Social Interaction
  (investing in healthy relationships)
- ☐ Mental Stimulation/Exercise
  (puzzles, reading, creative activity)
- ☐ Emotional Balance
  (dealing with anger, anxiety, or other emotions)
- ☐ Other:______________________

New Week
Scripture Meditation

For The Week Beginning / /
Day 1 of Week 5

**Psalm 139:17-18 NIV: How
precious to me are your
thoughts, God! How vast is the
sum of them! 18 Were I to count
them, they would outnumber the
grains of sand—when I awake,
I am still with you.**

Visualize the verse(s). What do the verse(s) speak to you, what emotions or memories do they invoke? What story do they tell or remind you of? What is God saying to you through the Scripture(s), and what can you speak back to Him?

This Week's Prayer & Reflection

For The Week Beginning / /
Day 1 of the Week

Heavenly Father, today, the first day of my week, I think of your care for me. I place my week into your caring hands.

Psalm 139:17-18 NIV: How precious to me are your thoughts, God! How vast is the sum of them! 18 Were I to count them, they would outnumber the grains of sand—when I awake, I am still with you.

This Week: In the Father's Care

Psalm 139:17-18 NIV: How precious to me are your thoughts, God! How vast is the sum of them! [18] Were I to count them, they would outnumber the grains of sand—when I awake, I am still with you.

Cares I'm Casting This Week

Coworker I'm Praying For

Patient I'm Praying For

I'm Grateful For

This Week's Shift Schedule

For The Week Beginning / /

Sunday	
Monday	
Tuesday	
Wednesday	
Thursday	
Friday	
Saturday	

To Dos

- [ ] ____________
- [ ] ____________
- [ ] ____________
- [ ] ____________
- [ ] ____________
- [ ] ____________
- [ ] ____________
- [ ] ____________

Weekly Self-Care Goal

One "self-care" thing I can do this week is . . .

Daily Scripture & Prayer

Date / /

John 14:27 NIV: Peace I leave with you; my peace I give you. I do not give to you as the world gives. Do not let your hearts be troubled and do not be afraid.

Thank you for peace. Thank you for protection. Thank you for patience for my patients.

Today's Reminders & Shift Notes

Shift Notes

To Dos

- [ ]
- [ ]
- [ ]
- [ ]
- [ ]
- [ ]
- [ ]
- [ ]
- [ ]
- [ ]
- [ ]
- [ ]

Daily Scripture & Prayer

Date / /

Hebrews 13:4-6 NIV: Keep your lives free from the love of money and be content with what you have, because God has said, "Never will I leave you; never will I forsake you." [6] So we say with confidence, "The Lord is my helper; I will not be afraid. What can mere mortals do to me?"

Thank you for peace. Thank you for protection. Thank you for patience for my patients.

Today's Reminders & Shift Notes

Shift Notes

To Dos

Thanks & Share

FROM THE CHRISTIAN *creatives* JOURNAL©

Thanks again for getting your copy of the Caregiver's Journal. Be sure to:

- **Leave us a great review.**
- **Order next month's journal.**
- **Check out our other titles,** including journals for Christian:
  - Caregivers and Nurses
  - Poets, Songwriters, and Spoken Word Artists
  - Praise and Worship Leaders and Musicians
  - Fashion Designers
  - Interior Designers and more
- **Join our email list for updates on new journals at:**
  - Purposehousepublishing.com

Made in United States
Troutdale, OR
11/03/2026

56844518R00050